It's Not Magic

*What I've learned in
70 years of
weight gain and loss*

by Susan Bonser

ISBN-13: 979-8812289980
Imprint: Independently published

Write to us at
susan.bonser@gmail.com

Other books by this author:
Penn journal of everyday life
Hands & Minds, David Gil's Bennington Potters
Life with Cushman, A Cushman Colonial Creations Memoir

http://thebonsers.com

Table of Contents

Intro

I am not a doctor. I hold an earned doctorate in education, but I am not a medical doctor. I state this at the start because I want to make clear that I am not prescribing for the reader anything that might affect their health and well-being. It is the reader's responsibility to consult their personal physician before undertaking any form of diet, exercise, and weight loss or weight gain regimen.

My goal here in this text is to share my personal experience and what I have learned over my seventy years of gaining and losing weight. The reader might find something of interest that they wish to incorporate into their own weight strategies (after discussing it with their doctor) or something they might wish to avoid based on my experience. In any case, I offer my experience to the reader as my opinion, based on years of trial and error and learning about myself.

And that is probably one of the most important conclusions I have drawn from my experience. No one can lose weight or maintain weight or cause me to gain weight for me. These are decisions and actions I take for myself. Or not. I control what food goes in my mouth. At times, I may eat for comfort or in celebration or for the pure joy of eating something delicious. But it is my decision to account for it, to balance the rest of my day's intake. It is my responsibility to get up out of my chair and move.

So, how did I get so empowered? I stopped listening to advertising. Ads are just trying to sell me something. I don't adopt silly sayings like, "Thin feels better than food tastes." I read that Kate Moss later regretted saying that. I take a no-nonsense, logical approach. It's work, but I am motivated to do the work to get the result I want. One thing I have learned about myself is that I have to work at it. I cannot be mindless about my health or I will not be happy. And at the bottom of all of this is the idea that I want to be happy, to feel good, to be healthy. So how did I get here? I will start at the beginning.

First Memories

Thinking back to memories I associate with weight and eating, there are good and bad recollections. They are all tied together, so it is impossible to pick out individual experiences that may have led to what eventually manifested as a feeling of pain associated with food or weight. This is the problem with food; it is so pleasant. Food is so tied to the people, culture and experiences of life. If the experiences are good, that good feeling becomes associated with the food and likely stays linked throughout a lifetime. My mother's Christmas morning rolls are my most vivid example. They were a fancy braided ring of iced sweet bread studded with raisins, candied citron and nuts. She made them every Christmas and served them warm with coffee as the snack while the children opened presents. What could be a happier memory than Christmas morning? I made the Christmas morning rolls years later for my own family and gifted them to my co-workers. Off-season, I found I was attracted to Entenmann's coffee roll, which bore a marked resemblance to my mother's Christmas morning roll. It's no wonder I found the Entenmann's cake a comfort. Of course, linking a food to a happy experience didn't automatically mean I was going to eat myself to death on it. The fact simply becomes a point of interest in examining my relationship to food. There is little doubt I found great comfort and excessive calories eating too many of the Entenmann's rolls over the years.

Even though I was a beefy baby, my first memory of feeling self-conscious about being overweight was when one of the boys who lived next door to us in Dunkirk, New York started

to refer to me as "whale". When I phoned his house and asked
to speak to one of his sisters, Karl would scream, "Whale's
on the phone" and then drop the receiver. It was one of those
experiences that sent a little shock through my body and stuck
with me for life. It's odd to look back now. I liked Karl. The
way he treated me was hurtful, so I just stayed away from
him. He was the oldest of four children. Karl's life shattered
when his mother committed suicide a few years later. I read
in the newspaper that he ended his own life when he reached
about the same age that she was when she died. He taught me
a valuable lesson. Who was hurting more? Was it Karl or me
from the way Karl treated me? I think it was Karl since I am
still alive. Still, when I was setting up passwords recently one
of the questions was, "What was your childhood nickname?"
I had to authenticate my account with a live person and the
representative asked me that question. When I responded,
"Whale," she was silent for more than a beat. She was probably
trying to imagine how that could be a positive nickname. It's
not. It's just a fact.

That neighbor family was composed of skinny and active
kids, living on food now considered Mediterranean. Their
father was Lebanese and meals often included homemade pita
bread, stuffed grape leaves (we called them cigars) and lots
of vegetables. Pita bread was torn and used to grab the pieces
of meat and vegetables. I loved eating over at their house and
watching the women gather weekly for baking. It was my first
taste of Baklava. When I left home, my mother gave me her
cherished recipe box with pre-printed file card dividers. There
were no recipe cards from her in the category of vegetables.
At the time we laughed about it. In my own life, I came to love

vegetables and to explore cooking with them in many ways. But simply adding vegetables to my diet was not a sure way to solve my weight problem, real or imagined.

My grandmother made some of my clothes, but my first really embarrassing clothes recollection was when my mother started to buy dresses for me from Chubbettes. I was in third grade so it was around 1960. I have since looked back at the company and their advertising. "Your chubby lass can be the belle of her class." At the time, apparently, in regard to clothing, heavy girls were termed chubby and boys were husky. An even more remarkable feature of this clothing line was that they offered parents a booklet titled, "Pounds and Personality, Advice for parents of chubby girls" to help them understand the "problems, talent development, shyness, tactless remarks, the 'game' of dieting, etc." This booklet was written by Dr. Gladys Andrews of the New York University School of Education. I would love to talk to her today. I wonder if she ever regretted being part of the Chubbettes business. The irony is that at the same time I was wearing Chubbettes, I was playing with my "ideally" proportioned Barbie in her perfectly luxurious Dream House. It was a double whammy.

I found a copy of the "Pounds and Personality" booklet recently. I bet that my mother read it and I wondered what advice she was given for her chubby little girl. A lot of the booklet text leaned into the idea of making the most of positive attributes. Such a pretty face. At one point, Gladys Andrews advises, "Do not be alarmed by nicknames such as Slim, Fatso, PeeWee, Chubbs, which go with growing up—they are friendly terms." Name-calling might go with growing up, but it is definitely not friendly. Her pronouncement makes me think that Andrews must have been a skinny child.

When I was about eleven years old, my mother signed me up for Mrs. Heil's dancing school. It was held in a ballet studio, so there were walls of mirrors. Once the steps were mastered, we participated in an evening of dance at the local country club. I wore a black velvet dress, no doubt manufactured by Chubbettes. I was paired with a husky red-headed boy named Mark Kuhner. When we discovered that the prize for winning each round of dancing was chocolate Ice Cubes, we became super-motivated to dance well. I remember winning the cha-cha portion of the evening. Like so many other times in my life, I don't remember anything else about the event but the dress, the boy, and the achievement. I often saw Ice Cubes at a candy counter years later and bought them, savoring the joy of victory again.

All of this provides some background to my childhood self-awareness and leads to my first memory of dieting. It was an observation of my mother, wanting to lose weight to fit into a special dress for my brother's wedding. She was already a smoker, something women in those days did to control their eating. When she wanted to lose weight, she went on a liquid diet and used a product called Metrecal. It apparently tasted badly but she persevered and lost the weight to fit the dress. Years later, when I wanted to lose weight, I followed her example. At eighteen I started to smoke cigarettes. Then I used Slim Fast to lose weight. Of course, this set in motion a lifetime of what is called call yo-yo dieting. Gain weight, crash diet, repeat. Metrecal was taken off the market when a high number of deaths were reported. The dangers of tobacco were exposed and most people stopped smoking. But I came out of these early experiences with some strong ideas about weight and losing weight. If it sounds like I am blaming my mother, I do not really. Those were the times and the fads of those times. My mother used to say, "Oh, what we do to our children!"

As a teen, I recall wishing to be thinner. I bought all of the teen fashion magazines: *Teen, Seventeen.* Colleen and Molly Corby were my idols. I pasted their magazine pictures to my closet door. My mother signed me up for the Louise Boyka School of Fashion and Charm in Schenectady, New York. I remember the first advice I got from Louise was not to smile so that my gums showed because it made me look like a horse. (So now I have a horse and a whale as my kindred spirits.) I tried to smile smaller. I also tried to become smaller. I kept off weight by drinking diet soda, Slim Fast and eating hard-boiled eggs and fat free yogurt. I played a lot of sports. I exercised on the living room rug. No more Chubbette dresses. My fitness goal was to ensure that boys I square danced with in gym class did not find a roll of fat at my waist. I wasn't fat, but when I wore a two-piece swimsuit to the beach at the lake I was uncomfortably aware of getting a lot of side eye.

I straightened my curly brown hair with Curl Free, ironed it, slathered it in Dippity-Do, then pinned it on soup cans in an attempt to be in style. I wore Ursula of Switzerland pants outfits. My reward was a bus trip to New York City to tour *Seventeen* magazine with Louise Boyka. I loved the offices and the work they were doing. I kept that idea at the top of my list as I made college and career decisions. I wasn't model-pretty, but then neither were the magazine editors I saw at

Seventeen magazine. I was smart, creative and motivated.
I started building my resume. I became editor of my high
school newspaper as a junior, something usually given to a
senior class member. I played on sports teams, was a football
cheerleader, and scorekeeper for our men's' varsity baseball
team. I got my working papers the minute I turned 16 and
landed a job at the local department store cosmetics counter
and decorating their display windows. I worked part time at
an apple farm store doing just about every job from baking to
hauling apples.

I chose Pratt Institute for college over Rhode Island School
of Design and Rochester Institute of Technology. My reason
was simple. I wanted to have as many teachers as possible
that were working professionals not professors. At Pratt,
especially if I took classes at night, my teachers were adjuncts
that worked real jobs during the day. They gave me practical
advice as well as freelance opportunities. I lived on $20 a week
to cover my school supplies and food. I waited tables in the
dorm café and worked in an office on campus. I played varsity
volleyball and in pickup volleyball after classes. I was as thin as
a rail. I let my hair go naturally curly. I entered a contest every
year of college, competing for a guest editorship at a big New
York fashion magazine. I was interested in the European travel
that went with the prize and in the opportunity to get a foot in
the door for a full-time job. In my senior year I won. I also got
the job.

To start with, I slept on the couch at work in the vice-
president's office. They would lock me in at night and let me
out in the morning. Once I had some money coming in, I got

an apartment. I soon discovered the anxiety that came with the big job. Fortunately, a girlfriend was at my apartment and recognized the symptoms when it happened. She handed me a paper bag to breathe into. I ate incredible New York deli sandwiches for lunch. I sampled extraordinary New York restaurants at lunch and at dinner. I joined the Museum of Modern Art. I also started to gain weight. At one time I made a concerted effort to walk, but mostly sat on a chair all the workday. My first landlord also owned a Brooklyn Heights bakery and would leave bags of pastries at my door at the end of the day. Nice, but really not helpful. The battle was on. I was on the road to a lifetime of weight loss and gain, of trying every new scheme that came down the pike to take off the weight. I will address them one at a time.

Gyms, Equipment, Exercise

I am not sure how many calories a person can actually burn at a gym but it never worked for me as a way to lose weight. Especially when I rewarded myself with a hamburger and cheese fries following a session. The first gym I joined was Jack LaLanne at Grand Central Station in New York City. It was conveniently located near my workplace but as a franchise it didn't last long. LaLanne was already a very old man, and people had pretty much forgotten him. When I was a child, my mother used to watch Jack LaLanne on the television. She also exercised along with a vinyl record to a tune called "Chicken Fat." Broadway composer Meredith Wilson who was famous for *The Music Man* wrote the song in 1962. It was sung by Robert Preston and had the same kind of high energy thumping beat as his renditions of *The Music Man* songs. *Chicken Fat* was produced for then President John F. Kennedy's Council on Physical Fitness. It was a jumping around, arm waving calisthenic routine. That vinyl record seemed as helpful as any session I had a Jack LaLanne. Other than initiate you on how to operate the equipment, the Jack LaLanne staff left patrons on their own. I remember the machine with the jiggling belt. One day, there was some sort of short in the machine and I got a shock from it. That was probably one of the last days I went to that gym. Over the long haul, I paid for a lot of gym memberships. I would use them for a short time, then stop but continue to pay for them — until I got tired of paying for nothing. I grew to favor certain equipment. For cardio, I liked the treadmill. I was interested in the raised desk and treadmill combination, but never got to the point of laying out the money for one before I blew out my

knee. A trainer had me lifting weights, but I never developed
good arm strength. I couldn't do a push-up to save my life.
I found stationery bikes boring, even though over the years
I bought a traditional and a recumbent bike for home. It's a
great place to hang laundry. I never took to spinning classes
or Internet services because I didn't care for someone yelling
dumb things at me to go faster or longer.

I took on a trainer at one of the gyms I joined over the years.
That worked for me. When he didn't have the certifications the
gym required, he trained privately and came to my apartment
mornings before work for an hour. I used to look out the
window to see if he had arrived and would spot him sitting
in his pickup truck smoking cigarettes. I crossed paths with
a lot of people in the fitness world that did not model the
behavior they promoted. Since all I had was hand weights, my
trainer devised a series of exercises that used my body weight
resistance to build muscle. It was actually a good way to train.
After a while he got his certification and went back to the gym.
I have joined a dozen gyms over the years. The factors that
probably affected how long I stayed was travel time, the quality
of the equipment, how busy the gym got, and finally cost.
Or bottom line, I just got bored with the routine. It was also
important who the clientele were. Macho jerks, male or female,
made a gym un-fun. I didn't see workouts as a competition. My
goals were to feel good, wear clothes comfortably, and have the
energy to be able to do other things.

I bought a Nordic Trak cross-country ski machine. I kept it
in my bedroom at the foot of the bed. Again, I used it for a
while and then started hanging laundry on it. The monotony

of the ski machine was mind numbing. I got rid of it. Many years later, I worked part time at a resort and was able to borrow actual cross country skis and poles to take home and use on the grounds of my apartment. This was fun for a short time. Eventually, even outdoor cross-country became circular. I stopped borrowing them. In spite of growing up in snow country, I was not a big fan of being cold. Maybe it was because I wore glasses and they would fog and ice up when I went skiing as a kid. Or it could have been the fall I took and limped for weeks. I bought a bicycle, thinking that getting outside and actually going somewhere might be fun. A friend talked me into a piece of equipment that was way too complicated. It had too many gears. It's not good to go for a bike ride and spend too much time looking down at the bike in order to operate it. The pleasure never quite kicked in for me. I sold the bike. Years later, I bought a bike rack for the car and a old time basic Schwinn to ride around Cape May at the Jersey Shore. It was pink and had a wicker basket to hold my shopping. My husband bought a blue one. It was the perfect bicycle. But then, of course, I lost flexibility of my knee after surgery and could no longer ride bikes.

Then there were the videotapes. Jane Fonda's is the first one I remember. Richard Simmons was a fleeting star and pleasant exercise companion on tape. Again, I did them a few times and got bored. I didn't have a lot of room in my apartment and most of the places I lived in New York City had cockroaches so I didn't relish time spent on the floor. As I lived in more normal apartments, I tried videos again and went through the same process of doing them a few times and then moving on. In fact, today I have a pair of DVDs sitting next to my television on movement for old people. I have had it six months and not broken the seal yet.

One man I dated was an avid kayaker. That sounded great to me, so I bought a kayak, roof rack, all the gear and took myself out on a nearby lake. Actually it was more like an hour's drive, but it was a beautiful winding road into the Pocono Mountains through woods and farms to get to the lake. I often put the kayak on my car in the morning and after work would drive up to the lake for a paddle. This is one piece of equipment that was a great success. I am not sure it contributed much to my fitness, aside from putting it onto and lifting it off of my car. But it was a spectacular way to unwind and enjoy nature. Which brings me to snakes. I do not like snakes. One day, getting the kayak into the water, a snake slithered alarmingly close to my legs. I stopped, frozen in the water and remember thinking, "OK, is kayaking over now? Does this kill it?" That incident did not, but shortly after, I was kayaking in a cove of the lake and encountered a slew of snakes. They got caught on my paddles. They tried to get into my boat. I battled to get out of there. Now I was done kayaking. I sold it on Ebay.

Though I stopped kayaking, I found once I was outdoors, I enjoyed jogging. I ran for three miles a day around the lake until I was about 55. Then my knee pain began to get in the way so I consulted a doctor who sent me to a specialist. I had an arthroscopic surgery and rehabilitation but my knee never came back. I stopped jogging; I couldn't even walk comfortably anymore. That is when the weight started to pile on because, of course, I didn't moderate my food to accommodate my lifestyle change. It was a disaster.

Weight Watchers

I start with Weight Watchers because that organization has, over the years, probably had the most influence on my weight life. My mother had a Weight Watchers book of recipes when I was a child. I don't remember that she ever joined or attended meetings, but I remember that book. Actually, I remember one recipe in that book: Zero Points Soup. It was a staple for her when she was dieting and it has become a staple for me as well. Basically, it is vegetable soup—carrots, celery, cabbage, tomatoes and vegetable broth. Like popcorn, it is one of the ways I got through my Weight Watchers dieting times.

The best part of the Weight Watchers design was that it was deemed a nutritionally sound diet by experts. There are two aspects to eating for weight loss. There is what you eat and how much you eat—the quality of your food intake and the quantity. Weight Watchers addresses both equally. It was not one of the hundreds of other crazy diets that have come down the pike that focus on a single food or food group. I tried most of them. I ate only cabbage, grapefruit, high protein, low carbohydrate, or vegetables for meals. I first joined Weight Watchers to lose my baby weight and took off some of the forty pounds I had gained. I joined again and lost more than 125 pounds just before I retired. While the plan changes at least slightly each season, there are some things I learned there that I feel worked for me over the long run —and some things that did not.

Weight Watchers uses a points system. They assign a certain number of points to each food and portion. You need their book or database subscription to track your food intake. That is a good business for them. It generates revenue by selling their books and subscriptions, but I don't feel like it served me well in the long run. Now, you can look up the Weight Watchers mathematical formula and apply it yourself to your food. You can also use one of the free Weight Watchers conversion calculators on the Internet. Why make extra work or expense. I needed to accurately gauge my food intake. That meant I needed to easily look up and track calories.

While Weight Watchers also offered a plan with a food list that required no tracking (I tried it) again I felt like I wasn't learning anything that would help me in the long run. The last time I did Weight Watchers, there were free foods. Fruit was a free food, so I lived on fruit. My opinion is that this was taking me back into the realm of crazy food diets not building a life skill. As soon as I reached my goal weight and stopped the plan, my weight started to go up again. This is, I understand, what happens to just about everyone.

Exercise or activity was also part of the Weight Watchers points plan. I could earn points for activities, which meant I could trade activity for food. Again, they prescribed the activity and point assignment, which I had to look up in their database. Later I adopted another, more meaningful understanding about activity and food that I did not get from this part of the Weight Watchers plan. I found on Weight Watchers that I was exercising too much, eating too much of the "free" foods, losing weight but not building a life skill that I could maintain. For me, this all got way out of whack. Using Weight Watchers points instead of actual units of measure kept me from understanding and planning to succeed in the long run. By the way, there is no free food. Comics tout celery as having negative calories, but other than water that may be it for free food.

What I found most helpful about Weight Watchers was their meetings. At that time, I could attend as many meetings in a week as I wanted—and I often attended multiple meetings. I went to the meetings, bought cookbooks and Weight Watchers snacks in the shop. I was given something to collect and take home—a recipe or a motivational idea. Today they have discussion groups online which I find totally useless. In fact, I have signed up twice in recent years for the online WW to have access to the tracking and database but found the rest of it was just not helpful. I am really not interested in Facebook-like postings of whining, bravado, chirpy words of support. I cringed when I logged in and the home screen announced, "Susan, you're better than bubble wrap!" Weight Watchers meetings were led by interesting people who had been through the program successfully. While their talks were prescriptive and felt canned by corporate, the physical act of removing myself from my stressful environment at work or at home gave me a change to breath, focus and renew my desire to lose weight. I would drive to different meeting places in nearby towns. I needed to remove myself from my environment to assess my progress and behavior in order to make modifications. At the time, this was not something I could do in my home or workplace. I was sorry when meetings became less and less available. I also understand that as a business model meetings are expensive. Meetings require a location to be rented, lights, cleaning and staff to support it. As the world became more social online, Weight Watchers corporate probably thought they could save a lot of money by limiting or eliminating physical meetings and replacing them with online resources. For me personally, it just doesn't work. But then, I am old. I do a lot of things online although human support is not one—unless there is no other way to interact. I still go to the doctor's office.

I kept the concepts I learned at Weight Watchers that were successful for me, and used them again long after I reached my goal weight. First was tracking. It is a lot of work to track food intake and it only worked if I was honest and accurate. But there is no better way I have found to actually change eating habits and lose weight. Weight Watchers gave me a booklet each week to track in. Since then, when my weight crept up I have tracked by handwriting in a journal, tracked online in my own documents or other free software or apps. At one time, I got tired of writing everything down and simply photographed my meals but that didn't work as tracking. I had to know the measures and calories in order to effectively track to get results. Tracking also provided a way, if I was not losing weight, for the leader to examine my intake and make corrections. Now, you may say that your sister-in-law is as skinny as a rail and doesn't track. Absolutely right. Some people know instinctively or have learned what to eat and how much—and when to stop. Whatever they are doing works for them without tracking. I have discovered through Weight Watchers that I am a person who needs tracking. I have to do the work to affect change.

The second concept I discovered at Weight Watchers, which

I found that I needed, was accountability. Once a week I went to a meeting, I stepped on the scale and my weight was written down. I received sticker stars and kudos for goals and successes, but more importantly I was accountable and received acknowledgment. The group celebrated big losses during the meetings. Software alone does not provide legitimate or effective accountability. For me, it requires interaction with other people—group leaders, doctors, an authority I value. I need a human being at the other end of the process. It entails a willingness to be judged which requires the judgment of a person whose experience and knowledge I respect. For me, this is not something that happens in a random online discussion group with strangers. A weight loss plan with built in accountability prevents me from floating off the plan like a helium balloon over the horizon. Once a year, my general practitioner's hospital has a 10-week weight loss online event. I participate but there is no accountability. In fact, my doctor may not be receiving this information in my chart because he has never mentioned it. There is no feedback loop with this weight loss event. There is no accountability. In fact, I have found that most weight loss schemes, plans, gimmicks do not have accountability built in. They simply hand you a diet, some articles to read and a way to track and then you are on your own. The Mayo Clinic Diet seems to be exactly this kind of plan. There is no accountability. When I got those goofy messages from WW online about bubble wrap instead of meaningful, relevant feedback, I knew I was in the wrong plan.

The most memorable takeaway from my Weight Watchers experience was one of my leaders explaining how she sometimes got to the point where she couldn't track or diet or exercise one more minute. She called it her "Screw it" moment which usually led to chocolate cake or other indulgence. Once it was over, she explained that she would recover and get back on track. I knew the feeling and I have heard "screw it" in my head many times over the years. I suspect that it means I am doing something that is too restrictive and feel I am making too great a sacrifice, so it is also a warning to examine my strategy.

Specialists & Seeking Help

There are a lot of people, doctors and companies out there who would love to convince the public that they have the magic key to losing weight and keeping it off. And they will gladly impart that knowledge to us in exchange for a fee. If we just eat their special food, drink their special drink, take their special pill, all of our weight problems will be a distant memory. I haven't fallen for every con out there, but I have done a few and I am here to tell you that there is no magic to weight loss or maintenance.

My first experience with what was humorously called a fat farm was when I was the art director of *Self* magazine. I wanted a vacation, a get-away, where I could get healthy. I chose a place in the mountains of Vermont, packed up my bicycle and leotards and took off. It was expensive, but at that time I could afford it. Looking back now, I would recommend going to a fat farm as a vacation. The only down side was that I was not prepared to find a few people who were seriously unhappy with their physical being and the program really did not address it. This program skimmed along the surface and gave women (it was all women when I attended) a place to get away and lose a few pounds without having to worry about work or the dishes or other household matters.

I didn't have a lot of weight to lose. In fact, when I went to one of the exercise classes, another client said in a loud whisper, "I just want to look like her." I stayed for a month and lost about twenty pounds. It was really easy to do this in a restrictive environment but I am not sure that has value in the long run.

The only thing I took away from the experience is that no one should eat a sandwich with more than one slice of bread. I still hear that proclamation in my head when I approach a sandwich all these years later. I have eaten many sandwiches with two slices of bread following my fat farm experience. Cute rules are entertaining but they don't mean much in the long run I have found.

My days at the fat farm were prescribed. We rose at a certain time, exercised according to a schedule and all of the guests' food was prepared specially and served in a dining hall. There was no thinking involved on my part. I just followed along like a lemming. Occasionally I would leave the pack and go for a bike ride. It was fall and it was beautiful in Vermont. I remember buying apples at a farm stand. No one could begrudge me an apple. Or was it just a form of rebellion, that I could eat something outside the prescription. You can see this might not have been a completely healthy experience for me emotionally.

The Vermont place was not the kind of fat farm where you might get a massage or a sauna. It was a building with dorm rooms and exercise rooms and a dining hall. It was a kind of bare bones vacation. Over the years, I have used my vacation time to ride horses at dude ranches in the Arizona desert and at Lake George, New York. I have rented an RV and camped by a lake in the Adirondacks. I got a Eur-rail pass and traveled Germany, staying at hostels and guest-houses. To be perfectly honest, the fat farm was really just another kind of vacation. It didn't have any long lasting value to my health or well being. It was a work break with health benefits.

The first doctor I went to who specialized in weight loss, put me on a liquid diet and diet pills. The liquid diet was Medifast and the pills were phentermine. I drank black coffee and, other than one limited meal a day, drank a thin liquid flavored like chocolate. I was given a screw-top container to mix the powder with water. It worked like magic and the weight fell off. My mother used to joke that I looked like a balloon that someone punctured and the air came out. But it wasn't the Medifast that was responsible for the weight loss. It was the pill. It was euphoric. My heart raced and I was happy. I worked on a computer and found I was exceptionally focused. This all felt very familiar so I got in touch with a cousin who worked in the pharmacological industry. He wasn't familiar with the drug but to me it felt just like the speed I would take once in a while at college to pull all-nighters during finals. Unfortunately the work I produced wasn't as spectacular in the morning after I crashed. I lost a lot of weight but as soon as I stopped the pills and liquid diet it all came right back and more.

The next doctor I chose to help me lose weight was a specialist in addictive behaviors. I thought that perhaps this might be the key. But when he prescribed my program I was surprised to find that there was no therapy component. I inquired about it but he told me "Don't go there." His plan was Medifast and two pills: phentermine and fenfleuramine, colloquially referred to as phen-fen. It was even more effective that the single drug that was previously prescribed with Medifast. Once again, I looked like a balloon that the air escaped from suddenly. I made weekly visits to his office for check up and refills. Then he died suddenly from lung cancer as a result of smoking. My addictive behavior expert died from smoking.

It's Not Magic 27

Programs developed around liquid diets and drugs were a response to the need for weight loss that was easy and fast. I didn't have to think. I didn't have to count or track or plan in any way. It was easy and it was mindless. I didn't learn anything. I didn't change my behavior. There was no discussion of nutrition or exercise. I have since learned that behavior modification is not easy or fast. In fact, if a program or product uses that terminology I know to stay away. I have learned by doing—and been lucky that I didn't hurt myself.

That was my last intervention by a doctor in my weight loss. A few years ago, a cousin got the lap band surgery and almost immediately began looking for ways to cheat it. She found ways around it and lost no weight in the first year that I noticed. Her behavior certainly was not modified. I look now at any of the plans, pills, surgeries on the market with a great deal of skepticism. To me, they all seem to be a scheme just to part me from my money. None would actually solve my long-term weight loss. My conclusion is that I have to do it myself. As easy as it was to lose weight by taking drugs, it turned out that at least one of the pills caused heart damage. I had to go for screening and was fortunate to find that I had not hurt myself by taking those drugs. As good as they worked, I would have to stay on them forever to benefit from their effect. Since I did not have any other health problems to justify that, why would I take that risk?

Books & Gurus

Over the years I have purchased hundreds of cookbooks. Many of them are published by Weight Watchers, but they also include natural, organic and vegetarian foods cookbooks and books by authors about nutrition. Of course, who needs to buy recipe books anymore with an Internet full of exceptional recipes. My favorite places to download recipes are the *Food Network, Bon Appetite, Food & Wine* and the *New York Times.* I look to Pinterest for creative ways to plate and tablescape. I avoid Martha Stewart. I have invested the time and ingredients in a few of her pretty recipes and they failed, so I don't go there anymore.

My most recent cookbook purchases have been from Jamie Oliver's kitchen. I love his attitude and his food so I enjoy his books. We first saw him on public television, making a plea for better school lunches in America. He made a convincing case and we hoped he would have an impact. But it seems the bureaucracy was victorious. Government subsidized food won. Cheese sticks and French fries for everyone. Parental pressure kept sugary chocolate milk on the menu.

The Jamie Oliver books I liked best were based on vegetables. I also watch his cooking show, *15-minute Meals* on DABL Not that I am in a big crunch for time, but the food is interesting and he is charming. I love that he uses fresh ingredients, grows herbs on the greenhouse porch. My favorite recipe of his is the caramelized red onion tart. Made in a cast iron pan, it starts out on top of the stove then goes into the oven to bake. I never had an onion tart before I made his.

Like Jamie Oliver, we raise herbs and greens on our porch. It makes a tremendous difference to the taste of foods to have fresh herbs at hand. We have raised basil, thyme, rosemary, cilantro, parsley, and a variety of lettuces and kale in a tall hydroponic garden with grow lights and sunlight. There are all kinds of hydroponic kits out there. Since my husband is an engineer, he started out with a kit then modified it to his liking. In the outdoor garden, we grow blueberries, tomatoes, peppers, potatoes, asparagus, dill, and mint. We grow in the ground, in raised beds and in fabric bags. We can what ripens and is more than we can use at the moment. Our favorite meal from the porch starts with basil pesto.

My latest nutritional expert's book is Dr. Michael Greger, *How Not To Die* was a catchy title. I passed it on to my son's partner. *How Not To Diet* then captured my attention and I also bought the subsequent recipe book that he produced alongside it. Those two books I kept and re-read periodically for inspiration. Greger relies on a lot of research crunching to come to his conclusions and recommendations about food and health. In general, my response to experts is: I hear a hundred things, I try ten, I incorporate one into my life. I don't ever really follow any of the advice prescriptively but rather find things in them that interest me and work for me.

From Dr. Greger, I have incorporated turmeric into my daily routine. I take a supplement and put turmeric onto food when it is served or into food as I cook. It's tasty, it's pretty and according to Greger it packs a punch for your health without any side effects. That means there is no known danger of overdosing or hurting yourself by putting too much on your plate. According to Dr. Greger's research and experience, "the single most anti-inflammatory food is the spice turmeric, followed by ginger and garlic, and the most anti-inflammatory beverage is green or black tea. The two most anti-inflammatory food components are fiber and flavones." (107-108). Of the hundreds of things I read in Dr. Greger's books and on his website, that one sentence represents what I took from it all and incorporated into my life. Tumeric, ginger, green tea and fiber comprise food habits that make sense to me and that I have successfully incorporated into my daily life. Someone else may read his work and come away with an entirely different set of food strategies—because there are so many in his work. But this is what stuck in my mind and what was easy for me to make a daily habit. I cook with ginger, fresh and powdered. I put ginger in my green tea. I love foods with lots of fiber like brown rice, nuts, legumes, leafy green and cruciferous vegetables. Greger made a reminder list, the *Daily Dozen*, which he also produced as a free app to check off each day. It is not really a tracker, but a reminder to add these things to your food intake.

Other meals that we have adapted from Dr. Greger's recipes are black beans and rice, mixed beans soup, hummus served with whole grain crackers or crudité. We are not religiously following Dr. Greger's food prescription, but we have incorporated a good deal of it into our previous food routine. We still like a steak off the grill or an egg once in a while. We eat fish and chicken more than red meat. We eat chocolate and sugary desserts in moderation. Dr. Greger strongly recommends a vegetarian lifestyle.

Probably our single most favorite recipe Dr. Greger recommends is his breakfast porridge he calls BROL, which stands for barley groats, rye berries, oat groats and black lentils. (556-557). We combine ½ cup of each grain plus 2 tablespoons of ground flax seeds with 4 ½ cups of water. We cook it in an Instapot by pressing the "porridge" button, which takes about 20 minutes. When it is done, we might add a little honey, fresh or dried fruit for sweetness and sunflower seeds for crunch. We like it so much that we buy the grains bulk from an organic producer and pack the dry mixture, measured out and ready to cook in small ZipLoc bags kept in the freezer. In the morning, all we have to do is empty a bag into the Instapot, add water and press the button. By far, this is my most favorite recipe from the Greger books.

Dr. Greger also recommends taking apple cider vinegar (the kind with the mother in the bottle). This was something we were already doing because our family doctor recommended it a few years ago. My husband remembered as a child that his grandfather took vinegar every day. We put a tablespoon into a glass of V-8 juice and drink it with our supplements every morning.

What I Have Learned

I have lost and gained weight for seventy years while reading, attending, joining and finding help. There are some lessons I have learned that I incorporated into my strategies now for losing and maintaining weight. Those things that I did that were not successful have been re-examined and discarded. Those concepts that worked were culled out and kept. Here is the result.

Number 1: Math

Losing and gaining weight are not magic. It is not mystical. There are no quick solutions. I am sorry if that disappoints you, I find it empowering. There are a lot of companies out there hawking all kinds of solutions with promises of fast, easy, painless, magical weight loss. It's baloney.

Weight loss for me, a relatively healthy person not on any medications, is simply math. I burn a certain number of calories each day and I eat a certain number of calories each day. If those numbers match up, I maintain my weight. If those numbers do not match up, then I either lose or gain weight. Calories are the standard measure of energy—not points or any other artificial gimmick companies may cook up. I measure everything in calories.

It is that simple.

In order to lose weight, first I have to determine how many calories I burn each day. That is my metabolism. There is a mathematical formula based on my height, weight, age and activity level that results in a number that is roughly what I burn each day. That is my goal number.

Then I decide how fast I want to lose weight. I usually choose to lose one pound a week. Some people freak out at that low a number because we are all primed by advertising to think we can safely lose 100 pounds in a month or in two weeks. But that is not a realistic way to approach safe and healthy weight loss. I have found if I crash off that kind of weight, I live a lifestyle I cannot maintain so when I stop the weight loss it comes right back on.

To lose one pound a week requires me to eat about 3,500 less calories than I burn. That means I need to reduce my daily food intake by 500 calories. So if I am currently burning 2,400 calories each day, I need to reduce my food intake to 1,900 calories each day.

I found that there are calculators on the Internet to figure out how many calories I burn based on my body, age and activity. I also found that when I bought a FitBit, one of the calculations it produces when I set it up is how many calories I burn each week. Either way, I can now monitor and control my energy.

Number 2: Accountability

For me to be successful, I need to be accountable. There are many ways to do this. I find that I can keep a handwritten journal. At the top of the page, I write my weight and the golden number that is how many calories I burn each day minus 500. Then I use the page to track my food intake, being sure not to go over the number. I use free online calorie databases to figure out how many calories I am eating. I weigh my food so I know exactly how many calories to assign. Am I perfect? No. But when I don't leave the 500-calorie margin in my day's food intake, I know that I cannot lose that one pound at the end of the week. I don't panic, I just understand it. And I know that it will take a little longer to get to where I want my weight to be.

My favorite way to be accountable today is through my FitBit. I set it up and know how many calories I burn each day. I log my food through the FitBit app and can see how many calories I have used. I can see the number of calories I have burned on both the FitBit watch and the app. In addition to the calories, I can also monitor my intake of water and movement or exercise. The FitBit encourages me to get up and walk 250 steps each hour for as many hours each day as I set. It also monitors activity and includes the energy burned while it maintains a record of my heart rate. This is a lot of ability to account for those things that affect my weight and health.

If that sounds like too much work, it is not. What I have learned about myself over years of weight gain and loss, is that I need to track and I need a method of accountability. This goes back to my choice of title, *It's Not Magic*. For me, weight loss is mindful. There is no way to mindlessly lose weight over the long run. Someone else cannot do it for me. I have to do this for myself. When I do, I feel good about myself and I feel empowered.

None of this will work if I am not honest. Once in a while,
I have to remind myself of that. Weight loss is math and
if I fudge the numbers it won't work. I have to weigh food
honestly. I have to input data honestly and accurately. It just
won't work if I am not honest with myself. This is data driven
weight loss and maintenance.

Number 3: Food Choices

What I eat is important to my health, but it is not important
to the accurate recording of the data. A calorie is a calorie.
So I don't beat myself up about a chocolate cupcake, but I do
record it accurately. I might be hungry when I go to bed if I
didn't eat high quality food throughout the day. That in itself
is an incentive to work toward eating whole grains, vegetables,
fruits and drinking water each day.

I don't follow a prescribed diet. I shop for foods I enjoy that
fall within the guidelines of healthy eating. I eat a slice of pizza
once in a while. I eat a cookie or a piece of candy. What is most
important to my long term goals is that I accurately track it.
What is important to my long term health is that I eat more of
the foods considered healthy and less of those that are not.

Number 4: Movement

Movement is important. I think of that expression, "sitting is
the new smoking". I watch my FitBit to get me up and moving
around. I make a point of going out and walking in the back
yard every day and the grocery store once a week. Since I have
trouble with my knee, I can walk short times on the treadmill,

but I strive to use an arm machine five days a week to get my heart rate up for 15 minutes or more.

What I do not do is over exercise. I am not a temporary fanatic just to burn calories. Been there, done that, it didn't work. I am looking to live my life first and lose or maintain weight second. I don't want to do anything that is over the top that I won't do every day for the rest of my life. I have found that temporary exercise results in temporary weight loss.

Number 5: Motivation

What makes me want to do this routine? Clearly there are times that I do not want to do it. What is it that makes me commit to doing it? In the past, it worked for a short time that I had committed money to losing weight. For me, I just get tired of carrying extra weight and the burdens it creates. Sometimes, it is coordinated with a program from my doctor's office and sometimes it is just the January 1 tradition. My FitBit gives me daily motivation. But mostly, it is just that I want to feel my best. In my head and in my heart, it is my desire that drives me to do the work that I need to do to lose and maintain the weight.

I seem to have a set point, a weight number that I gain to and then hold on until I do something about it. It is a high number, so I have a real roller coaster history of ups and downs since I was a young adult.

When I was about 30 years old I contracted a disease that affected my eyes, my lungs, my joints and left me bedridden or in a wheel chair. Like all life experiences, there were some things I learned that stayed with me over the years since. One was that I am me, inside my body. I am not my body. I am the person inside. No matter how bad things were for my body during that time I was sick, I was still in there. So I have never taken much offense at people judging me who have not had that life experience. My value is not in the superficial physical body I am in. I am the person inside. Doctors cured my illness. I can fix my weight. There is nothing wrong with the me inside. I am a really special, happy, smart, funny person. No matter what my body is up to.

Some Final Thoughts

Get yourself a good scale to weigh yourself. Weigh yourself at the same time each day wearing the same clothing. Also get a good food scale. Measuring food in cups and teaspoons seems to me to be far less accurate and more involved than simply weighing food on a scale in ounces. Choose a food scale with a Tare function so you can put your plate on the scale and zero it out then start weighing the food as you add it to the plate.

Get rid of your old, large clothes as you lose weight. Donate them to a clothing bank if they are still in good condition. Don't keep a range of sizes of clothing in your closet. It makes it too easy to slip back. Move forward with the intention of staying forward.

I have to mention the skin problem with losing weight. Losing one pound a week might give my skin a better chance of catching up to the new size better than crashing off a hundreds pounds in a few weeks, if that is even possible. As I aged, I found my skin less resilient to the ups and downs. One of the things I did was to use loofa gloves religiously in the shower to stimulate my skin and remove dead skin. Also, since the time of my first pregnancy, I have used and continue to use cocoa butter and coconut lotion to minimize stretch marks and dry skin. At the very least it is a pampering gesture and smells nice. Though I don't go overboard any more on exercise, movement is important and resistance is helpful to me. They used to tell us, "Muscle burns more calories than fat." I just don't adopt those maxims any more. I do what makes me feel best. Activity, movement and resistance make me feel good.

If I am tracking and being honest and still not losing weight, then there are two things I have to consider. The first is that I may need to see my doctor. There are all kinds of physical reasons for weight movement or lack of movement and the doctor is the one to check them out. The second is that commercial nutrition information on food packaging may not be accurate. I have read that some calorie counts may be off as much as 20%. I know, that is disturbing. Companies may fudge the number of calories in their products. It's easy to understand why. They want to sell more. They want us to eat more. It's not going to happen.

I am in charge and I control my weight. There is no magic, but there are strategies to be successful. It starts with me. I have to figure out what works for me then put in the work to make it happen. If I don't, my son will be quoting this back at me some opportune moment in the future. He is a very kind person, but like all kids he remembers everything his mother says.

About

Susan and David Bonser are retired from the daily grind but enjoying being productive in their post nine-to-five lives. Susan had worked as a Madison Avenue art director, director of internet operations for an NHL team and tenured college professor. David had worked as a high efficiency energy engineer and started his own company to design and install geothermal heating and cooling units which he designed and built. They share a love of family, history, Pennsylvania, cooking, photography, football, DIY, and bringing old houses back to life. And publishing, of course. You can see more of the books and magazines that they publish at their web site: http://thebonsers.com.